READ THIS BEFORE YOU DIET

The Science of Weight Loss Explained

KIRSTEN BÉDARD

Illustrations by Bjoern Arthurs

Cormorant Books

The publisher gratefully acknowledges the support of the Canada Council for the Arts and the Ontario
Arts Council for its publishing program. We acknowledge the financial support of the Government of
Canada through the Canada Book Fund (CBF) for our publishing activities, and the Government of
Ontario through the Ontario Media Development Corporation, an agency of the Ontario Ministry of
Culture, and the Ontario Book Publishing Tax Credit Program.

LIBRARY AND ARCHIVES CANADA CATALOGUING IN PUBLICATION

Bédard, Kirsten, author
Read this before your diet : the science of weight loss explained / Kirsten Bedard.
Issued in print and electronic formats.

ISBN 978-1-77086-496-2 (hardcover). — ISBN 978-1-77086-497-9 (HTML)

1. Nutrition. 2. Food. 3. Weight loss. I. Title.

QP141.B43 2017   613.2   C2016-907290-8
                                        C2016-907291-6

Cover design: angeljohnguerra.com
Interior text design: Tannice Goddard, bookstopress.com
Illustrations by Bjoern Arthurs
Printer: Friesens

Printed and bound in Canada.

The interior of this book is printed on 100% post-consumer waste recycled paper.

CORMORANT BOOKS INC.
10 ST. MARY STREET, SUITE 615, TORONTO, ONTARIO, M4Y 1P9
www.cormorantbooks.com

For Papa Bear.

"It is only by selection, by elimination, by emphasis, that we get at the real meaning of things."

CONTENTS

Introduction

When I was sixteen years old, in grade eleven, I became interested in food and nutrition. I was working part time at the local branch of the Toronto Public Library and would often hide in the health section on my shifts, straightening the books, really scouring the pages. I absorbed everything I read on healthy eating and was convinced that a low-fat, high-carbohydrate diet was the way to go. This belief was solidified, of course, by the fact that I loved cereal and bagels, pasta and rice, and low-fat rice cakes and crackers.

Most days, after school, walking home, I would duck into the health food store to purchase sesame sticks or all-natural licorice. There I met Tony, a gentleman who worked at the store. Curious and forever trying to understand more about the things I had read, I was brimming with questions and confusions. What I learned from Tony, and then again ten years later, was the truth about carbohydrates, and why stable blood sugar is the foundation of good health.

During one of our chats, Tony asked me what I ate in a day. I relayed my low-fat, high-carbohydrate regimen to him. He shook his head. Then, for the next twenty minutes, I argued the merits of my eating. He humoured me by listening. Tony told me to cut back on carbohydrates and increase fat. "Drink a quarter cup of olive oil a day. Eat fish and nuts and seeds. Get rid of grains, refined or not. If you do, you'll see what changes come, mentally and physically." I was terrified, but did as he suggested.

He was right, of course.

Ten years later, at the age of twenty-six, having completed a degree in nutrition, and now working as a personal trainer and nutrition consultant, I met my second mentor, Mike. He was giving a talk on the psychology of sport. I was in awe of both his wisdom and his physical stamina — at sixty-five he could bounce up and down, doing one hundred consecutive jumping push-ups. Mike coached athletes. He himself competed in Ironman races.

At the time, I was an avid runner and had recently begun cycling, weaving my own training into long days of training others.

I called Mike after to ask if I could take a few coaching sessions. To this day, the lessons he taught me in our few meetings continue to be invaluable in both my own training and in my work.

I wanted to learn exercise strategies to increase my speed and my endurance, but Mike's first advice was to change how I ate. No grains, no sugar. He advised me to eat nuts, seeds, olive oil, fish, and greens. Eat fat for fuel. Sugar was only useful right before and during performance. (This all sounded rather familiar, though by now I had slipped gradually back into a higher carbohydrate regimen.) I took Mike's advice. My performance improved noticeably, and I also lost ten pounds. While I wasn't looking for it, the weight loss was an indication of how much better my body had become at burning both food and stored calories as fuel for energy.

Since Tony and Mike there have been a few more brilliant mentors. I went back to school at the age of thirty to learn physiology and pathology from a professor who taught her courses using visuals and vivid analogies to explain the brain and hormones in a way that connected all the dots. I finally understood the role the brain plays, and the way it responds to blood sugar via hormones and the endocrine system.

Weight gain has everything to do with the brain, as does weight loss. Instinctively, we all know that minimizing calories and exercising are two principles that are critical to weight loss, but the stabilizing of blood sugar was an epiphany for me. Stable blood sugar is the foundation for good health and fitness.

The science of food and the body became a lifelong passion. The more I understood how drastically eating and exercise affect everything in the body, the clearer my life's mission became: to coach and teach people how to eat better and why. I have been working in the field of nutrition and exercise for the last twenty years, consulting, teaching, and writing.

I firmly believe that education is the best way to prevent people from lurching from one diet to another, making it possible to have control over their weight and well-being. My intention is to clarify the complex science of weight loss according to three simple principles: stabilize, minimize, and exercise.

Following the three principles set out here leads to improved energy levels, mental capacity, physical performance, cholesterol levels, and blood pressure. It can also lead to permanent loss of excess weight.

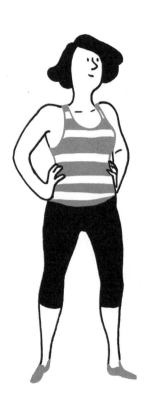

THE SCIENCE OF WEIGHT LOSS EXPLAINED

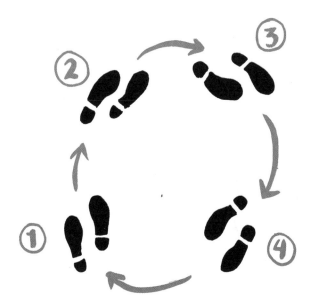

Do you feel like you keep going in circles, embarking on the journey to weight loss and improved health, full of optimism and determination, only to end up right back where you started?

You're not alone.

It's no wonder we chase our tails. Every day, we're bombarded by information and misinformation that mould our beliefs and justify our habits.

This has made losing weight — simply understanding how to eat — far more confusing than it has to be.

Do you want to lose ten pounds? Do you have Type 2 Diabetes, high blood pressure, persistent pain, chronic inflammation? Are your energy levels low and your moods even lower?

Regardless of why you want to lose weight, the way of going

about it is the same. And, contrary to what you may believe, it can be quite simple.

In this book, I'm going to teach you the three basic principles of weight loss:

1. Stabilize — balance blood sugar levels.
2. Minimize — reduce calorie intake.
3. Exercise — Move daily and build muscle.

All weight loss depends on these three principles.

Stabilize   Minimize   Exercise

How many diets have you tried and tossed aside?

Why do diets alone not work?

Whether you're an apostle of Atkins, a preacher of the Paleo, or a South Beach survivor, there is no shortage of diets. There are already thousands of health and weight loss books sitting on bookstore, library, and living room shelves everywhere. We don't lack information.

The problem isn't the diet.

It's two things. The first is that we obediently follow a diet for a defined period of time, thinking once we've lost those extra ten pounds, that we can go right back to our old ways.

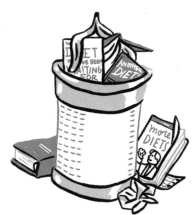

The second is that we don't understand the science behind the diet.

There are two ways we can approach weight loss. Only one of them works.

The first way is to blindly follow a diet — counting, measuring, and weighing. The weight will come off for a while — until we grow tired of the deprivation.

The second way is to learn about and understand the role our brain and endocrine system play in responding to and affecting how and what we eat. It comes down to three core principles. When we understand them, we can be strategic about weight loss, knowing not only what to do, but why we want to do it.

A successful strategy for weight loss is only possible if we know the science of food, how the body burns food, and, most importantly, how the brain oversees the process.

When we diet, we cut back on calories. This is a necessary component to losing weight as it is an excess of calories that causes weight gain, and so it follows that a deficit of calories will lead to weight loss. But actual weight loss, and maintenance of an ideal weight, depends on much more than a deficit of calories.

There is an intricate system at work within the body that affects our weight, our energy levels, and our state of health. There are numerous interconnected relationships between food, blood sugar, hormones, and the brain that determine what happens to the food we eat.

To focus solely on a deficit of calories does not take into consideration this highly sensitive system. In order to lose weight permanently — which is entirely possible — we must be savvy and strategic, which comes back to the brain.

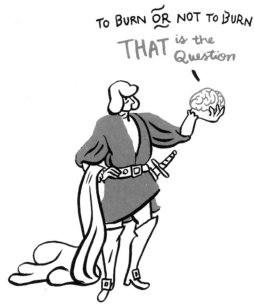

The Brain is Boss

The brain controls every thought, feeling, memory, physical movement, bodily function, and chemical reaction that takes place within the body. It also has the first and the final word when it comes to our weight and overall well-being.

No matter which diet we follow, it is the brain that decides what happens to the food we consume and to the stored calories we're trying lose.

If the brain approves of the way we eat, then we burn our calories as fuel. If it doesn't approve, we store those calories as fat. Together with the endocrine system, the brain is the boss of weight gain and weight loss. When we know how to align eating and exercise with brain chemistry, weight loss will not only be easy, it'll be permanent.

The trouble is that our heads are already full of information and misinformation. So, before we go any further, there's something we have to do first.

Clean the Slate

If we don't clean the slate, we'll set out on our mission to lose weight, get partway there, and then those saboteurs that hijack all weight loss and long-term health endeavours will block our path.

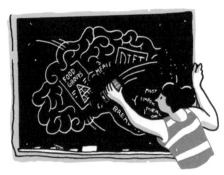

Much of our understanding about healthy eating has been spoon-fed to us by our parents and their parents before them. They pass down their wisdom mostly by example.

As adults, we acquire knowledge — or rather, information — about different foods from the very industries responsible for their production. Over the years, all this information takes root, gradually hardening into daily habits and firm-held beliefs.

Marketing, misinformation, and manipulation come at us from all directions, enticing us to want more, need more, buy more, eat more. We grasp diet trends because we want to be healthy, not just lose weight. It's hard to believe, but the very information that we put our trust in may actually be responsible for fattening us up.

Even more profound is how certain kinds of foods become the mainstay of our diets. All carbohydrates — whole and processed — are part of almost every meal and snack.

The problem is that the driving force of the food industry is at odds with the underlying motivation of the human brain. These interests don't align. One seeks wealth, the other health.

It seems we've lost the critical sense to distinguish foods that are profitable from those foods that are actually healthy and useful. Unless you have your own farm, most of us are at least partially dependent on the food industry for our nourishment, but if we're also seeking to improve our well-being, it's essential that we question what, how, and why we're eating.

It's time we became more mindful investigators.

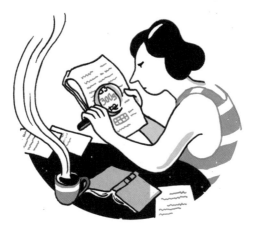

Unmasking Carbohydrates

Here's some straight talk about carbohydrates. Following the three principles is only possible if we have an awareness and understanding of exactly what carbohydrates are and how they impact blood sugar, the brain and the endocrine system, and our weight.

No other food presents us with as great a dichotomy as carbohydrates. Loved and loathed, they are equally healthful and harmful. Their "comfort" factor lures and hooks us, then fattens us up, making us sick. Whether we want to lose weight, boost energy levels, lower harmful cholesterol, or simply improve the state of our health, the first step is to unmask carbohydrates.

Beneath their whole-grain and high-fibre disguises, all carbohydrates are sugar. We're hooked on them. We can't get enough. They fill our minds, our diets, and our fat cells. They are our comfort, our comfort foods. We love them so.

The smallest serving of grains is comprised of hundreds of glucose molecules. Glucose is sugar. Now we can devise our own theories about whether this makes grains good or bad, or we can simply accept the science. All grains are densely packed with sugar, and when it comes to sugar's impact on health, one thing is for certain: less is always better.

Carbohydrates equal sugar

All foods — except meat, fish, eggs, cheese, butter, and oils — contain a little or a lot of sugar. Sugar is not only found in sweet-tasting foods. From cereal to legumes, bread to crackers, fruit to whole grains, to the most wholesome vegetable — they're all made up of sugar.

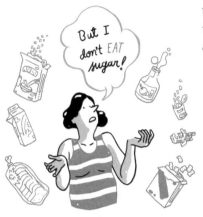

There are three simple sugars: glucose, galactose, and fructose. Glucose is our greatest concern, because it's the most pervasive in our diets, making it the trickiest one to get away from. Glucose is hidden in most of the foods we eat every day.

Do you remember the Potato Head toys? They were plastic potato-like dolls that came dressed in an assortment of hats, gloves, wigs, and glasses. When you pulled off their disguises, however, they were all the same! Glucose isn't much different.

No matter how the food industry dresses them up, all the whole and not-so-whole carbohydrates we consume are broken down in our intestines into their basic components: glucose molecules. They may come in a bright array of pretty packages, plastered with proclamations of bowel-energizing fibre, but all of them make their way into the bloodstream as simple sugars.

It comes down to chemistry

Unless we're walking across a continent, hiking the Himalayas, or working as a bike courier in a major city, many of us should cut back on carbohydrates, especially if we want to shed a few pounds and improve our health.

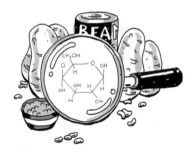

The trouble with carbohydrates is that they are full of sugar. And sugar can make us fat. Why? Excessive consumption of carbohydrates causes blood sugar to spike. The brain likes this feeling — for a few minutes — and then it panics. It calls on the hormone insulin to get that sugar out of the bloodstream, which it does by dumping it into fat cells.

The aftermath of this is low blood sugar, which also causes the brain to panic. This time it calls on another hormone, cortisol. Cortisol holds onto body fat and increases our cravings for sugar. Do you see how high and low blood sugar create a vicious cycle?

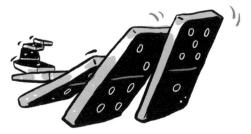

This cycle doesn't stop at simple weight gain. In time it leads to obesity, as well as high blood pressure, inflammation, decreased brain function, a weakened immune system, and heart disease. A high carbohydrate diet sets a dangerous domino effect in motion.

High carbohydrate foods — grains, pasta, oatmeal, bread, sweets, cereal, granola, and even fruit — can all lead to blood sugar fluctuations, namely high blood sugar.

High blood sugar leads to high insulin levels, which causes food to be stored in fat. High insulin levels cause two things: fat storage (weight gain) and, eventually, insulin resistance, where the body's cells no longer respond to insulin and blood sugar levels stay high.

Insulin resistance is associated with sex hormone alterations, namely conversion of estrogen to testosterone in women, which can lead to depression and polycystic ovaries.

Adrenal dysfunction is another manifestation of insulin resistance, as cortisol is constantly being released in response to the stress of all the sugar in the bloodstream and not in the body cells. Cortisol makes blood sugar levels higher, and eventually the adrenals tire of producing cortisol and they themselves fatigue, thereby pushing the immune system into overdrive.

Adrenal dysfunction and immune system overdrive cause increased inflammation throughout the body — pain, swelling, digestive troubles, infection, illness — which in turn affects the brain's neurotransmitters, and the brain itself becomes affected, resulting in lack of focus, decreased memory, and impaired cognitive function.

The brain, not working at its maximum capacity, then slows down the production of thyroid stimulating hormone, which lowers thyroid hormone production, and metabolism slows down. When metabolism slows, less energy is being produced within cells and therefore more food is being stored rather than burned and converted into energy. This leads to further weight gain.

The reduction in thyroid hormone also affects the liver and gallbladder, making them both sluggish, unable to flush cholesterol, triglycerides, and toxins from the body. This further impacts the immune system and increases inflammation. Along with this comes glycosylation — a process in which sugar molecules are added to protein, which results in stiffening of muscles, tendons, and joints, and is related to the damage evident in diabetes.

Does this mean that we should steer clear of all carbohydrates? No. Carbohydrates can be a useful form of fuel for the body, in smaller amounts and in less dense forms.

The trouble is that we eat too many of them, in all their forms, every day, all day long.

It is the cumulative sugar tally from all carbohydrate sources that perpetuates these problems. In order to lose weight and improve our health, it's essential to have a clear understanding of carbohydrates.

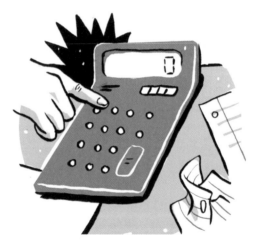

Success with weight loss begins with stable blood sugar levels

STABILIZE: THE FIRST PRINCIPLE

Imbalanced blood sugar makes us fat

Imbalanced blood sugar leads to weight gain, regardless of whether or not we're consuming too many calories. Many of us have come to believe that we lose weight by cutting calories, which is a reasonable assumption, though only partially true. Anyone who's tried to lose a few pounds by strictly counting calories knows that cutting calories is only part of the picture.

If we want to lose weight and keep it off, we must stabilize blood sugar levels before and above all else. Without balanced blood sugar, all weight loss efforts will eventually fail. If blood sugar spikes and drops all day, the pounds will stay where they are, or fall off and then reappear as soon as the cravings spike and we give in to them.

Remember: the brain gets the final word.

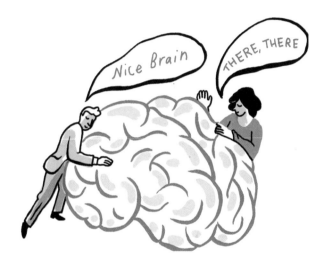

When the brain isn't happy with how we're eating, we'll know

We all believe we eat a healthy diet, and yet, the number we see on the bathroom scale keeps climbing, as if some invisible and growing creature is standing on it with us. We may be consciously and diligently dieting right now, counting every calorie and step taken, and we still may not be losing any weight.

The brain only allows us to lose weight if it agrees with not only how much we're eating, but what and when. Even on a calorie deficit, we can still be eating in a way that spikes blood sugar levels, and the brain will continue to store food in fat cells, with the help of its loyal defence squad, insulin.

The Insulin Police

Insulin is the body's Sugar Defence Team. Like a drug squad, insulin's primary aim is to defend the body's cells against the harmful impacts of excess sugar. How does it do this? It sweeps sugar out of the bloodstream and into fat

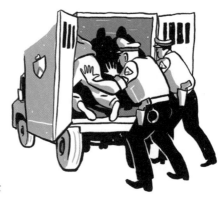

cells. When we continually eat glucose-dense carbohydrates and repeatedly spike blood sugar levels, the brain gets ticked off and insulin gets angry. When you tick the brain off too often, there's trouble.

When gangs of sugar — in every hidden, wholesome, whole grain combination — are racing around the body, insulin responds by corralling them and locking them up in fat cells. The more sugar (carbohydrates) we eat, the more calories get dumped in fat cells. But the trouble doesn't end there.

Our energy crashes. After insulin has removed sugar from the bloodstream to fat cells, blood sugar drops, since everything we just ate has been stored rather than burned. Low blood sugar isn't good either. What goes up must come down.

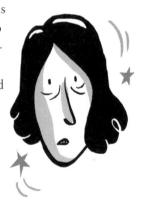

And what goes down must come up.

After insulin dumps all the fuel we just ate into fat cells, our blood sugar now drops down very low. For many of us, this happens after a hefty lunch. You know the feeling — as much as you may try to keep your eyelids open, they want to nap. Low blood sugar makes us feel wonky, dizzy, faint, unable to focus, irritable, moody, and consumed by cravings. Cortisol has arrived on the scene.

Cortisol

Similar to insulin, cortisol's job is to protect the body. There are two reasons why the brain calls on cortisol. One is in response to external stress, mental or physical. The second is in response to something internal, low blood sugar. It follows insulin when it clears up high blood sugar or it is activated as a result of long periods without eating. Both stress and low blood sugar are dangerous to the body since they cause essential processes to go awry or shut down. When blood sugar drops too low, often insulin's aftermath, the brain calls on cortisol to set things right. If insulin is the body's defence team against too much sugar, cortisol is the body's offence team when there's not enough. Cortisol's job is to elevate blood sugar in case we have to fight, or run fast. It does this by increasing sugar cravings.

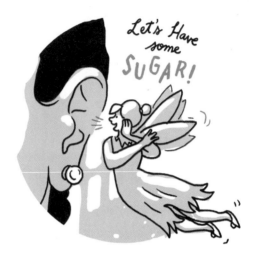

In the same way that Tinkerbell lured Peter Pan into all sorts of trouble, cortisol whispers in our ear, begging, "More sugar. Please!!!" It wants sugar and will do anything to get some, including luring us back into the exact same situation we've been trying to escape. For some of us, cortisol races around all day, begging us for more sugar in all its hidden forms. We're always hungry, never satisfied. Weight gain central.

Cortisol can't be reasoned with

Cortisol is like a tired, whining, hungry kid in the cereal aisle at the grocery store. When blood sugar is low, cortisol is relentless, kicking and screaming for more carbohydrates. "Something, anything, the more, the better!" it cries until we cave in, justifying our choices as necessary, wholesome, or natural. The problem is that every time we give in to it, we spike our blood sugar again.

Low blood sugar always follows high blood sugar, and cortisol always follows insulin. Don't give in to it. The way to deal with cortisol is to avoid it, and if you must, ignore it.

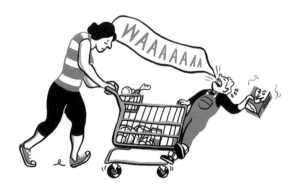

Turn Down the Volume

When you're feeling low or having a craving or longing, override the urge to reach for a bagel or a cookie. If you don't, you'll be right back to high blood sugar another insulin

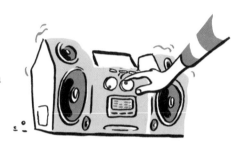

surge, and another crash. Don't end up back where you started, stressed and starved and fatter still.

Ignore the cravings. And when cortisol comes calling, cover your ears. We can't fix low or high blood sugar with more sugar. The problem is sugar! When we most want carbohydrates is precisely when we must work hardest to avoid them.

When blood sugar is constantly bouncing around, both insulin and cortisol will wreak havoc. They'll fatten us up, over and over again, year after year. They'll begin to make us sick.

Stable blood sugar is the first and most important principle of weight loss

If we're dieting by limiting calories, while still eating high amounts of glucose, the brain will panic and sabotage the weight loss endeavour yet again, as it has in previous attempts. When blood sugar is balanced, the brain is pleased. Stable blood sugar provides the brain with a sense of calm contentedness whereby it stops summoning fleets of insulin and cortisol.

When blood sugar is balanced — not spiking and not crashing — we can convince our brains to stop storing our food.

We can then minimize the calories we're eating, and the brain will begin to relinquish the fuel it has hoarded in fat cells.

The key is to tiptoe beneath the brain's panic radar. This means not overeating or undereating during any period of time, and eating small meals that are a balance of protein, fat, and less glucose-dense carbohydrates at regular intervals throughout the day.

There are six strategies for stable blood sugar:

1. Eat vegetables for carbohydrates
2. Counterbalance carbohydrates with protein and fat
3. Eat fat to win the fuel race
4. Don't jack blood sugar at breakfast
5. Eat snacks to keep steady
6. Don't let wine and other alcohol throw you off balance

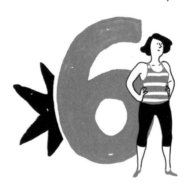

THERE ARE **SIX STRATEGIES**
FOR STABLE BLOOD SUGAR

1. Eat Vegetables for carbohydrates!

In order to balance blood sugar and lose weight, we must begin by reducing our carbohydrate intake. The smartest and simplest way to do this is to eat vegetables.

Even while losing weight, we always need some carbohydrates. The key is to be choosy about which ones. What we want is maximum nutrition for the least amount of sugar. Dense glucose carbohydrates — such as grains — are high in glucose and low in nutrients. They're the common culprit for most of us.

Vegetables get the vote in this campaign. The leafy green and cruciferous types, in particular, contain very small amounts of glucose, but are rich in fibre and water. They can be eaten leisurely, in large amounts, while still maintaining steady blood sugar and minimizing calories. Vegetables are, without question, the most sensible carbohydrate.

Bored of kale?

Here is a list of vegetables, but remember that the selection is endless:

Lettuces — leaf, romaine, head, butter, Boston, mesclun, radicchio, escarole, wild chicory, lambs, curly chicory, endives.

Cabbages — green, white, red, savoy, Brussels sprouts, kale, ornamental kale, bok choy, guy lan.

Ornamental — broccoli, cauliflower, artichokes, rapini.

Stalk vegetables — green asparagus, celery, Swiss chard, white asparagus, rhubarb chard, kohlrabi, palm heart, rhubarb, bamboo shoot, fennel, glasswort, cardoon.

Bulbs — white garlic, red onion, scallion, shallot, water chestnut, green onion, Spanish onion.

Fruit vegetables — green and red peppers, yellow peppers, tomatillo, cherry tomato, vine tomato, plum tomato, grape tomato, white eggplant, Asian long eggplant, Italian eggplant.

2. Counterbalance carbohydrates with protein and fat

Think of a tightrope walker trying to get from one end of the rope to the other without crashing to the ground. She uses a counterbalance to keep steady as she moves across the rope.

Carbohydrates (which we can think of as vegetables from now on) are like the tightrope walker travelling through the bloodstream towards the destination of fuel. Protein and fat act as the counterbalance. They help prevent both the spike and the crash. In this way, they ensure food is burned as fuel, not stored as fat.

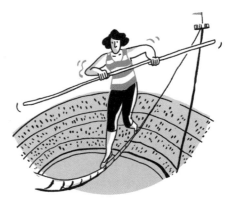

Protein and fat help to slow down the absorption of food from the intestines into the bloodstream. They temper the flow of sugar entering the blood, and in doing so, keep us off that insulin-cortisol roller coaster. Since they take longer to break down and get absorbed, protein and fat also satiate our hunger for longer periods, which is important for losing weight.

Protein is versatile

Protein is made up of amino acids that are linked together in food, and then broken apart during digestion, and later reassembled in the body as needed. While amino acids have numerous jobs, their primary role is to repair and rebuild all of our cells and tissues. Neither carbohydrates nor fats can perform the job of building and repair. During weight loss, while on a calorie deficit, protein is also highly versatile, and able to transform into whatever the body needs, including fuel for energy.

Everyone needs protein

The question is: How much? For the average person, three to six ounces of protein twice a day, along with a smaller amount in snacks, is more than enough. But when you think of protein, don't just think of meat. Aside from meat, other sources of protein include fish, eggs, cottage cheese, Greek yogurt, and pure protein powders.

What if you're vegetarian?

Many people choose not to consume animal products, but when it comes to weight loss, this can be tricky. There are two things to be cautious of if you're vegetarian. The first is that some of the amino acids in animal products are essential, meaning the body can't produce them on its own.

The greater concern, however, is that typical vegetarian or vegan meals — grains and beans — are loaded with glucose. Legumes, unbeknownst to many people, are among the most glucose-dense foods. If you're not convinced, read the nutritional label on a can of beans.

There are hundreds of glucose molecules in even a small amount of grains. A bowl of beans and grains isn't an ideal meal for stabilizing blood sugar. But don't be dismayed. With careful attention, vegetarianism and weight loss can pair well together.

We know that counterbalancing carbohydrates is high-priority, so if you are consuming a lesser amount of protein, you will want to increase healthy fats in order to keep your blood sugar levels stable.

Many vegetarians increase carbohydrates as a way to replace calories from pure protein. To stabilize blood sugar, they are better off increasing healthy fats, rather than large servings of grains and beans. Fuel instead with avocados, nuts, seeds, nut butters, and oils. Both protein and fat will counterbalance carbohydrates.

3. Eat fat to win the fuel race

Do you remember the tale of the tortoise and the hare?

The hare challenges the tortoise to a race. Reluctantly, the tortoise agrees. She doesn't much like to race. When the gun goes off, the hare bounds out in front, sprinting ahead, leaping

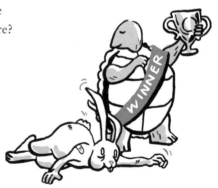

along until he crashes, not even halfway to the finish. Flat out of energy already, the hare lies down for a nap. The tortoise, on the other hand, moves along, smooth and steady, calm and consistent, past the dozing hare, and straight to the finish line.

Think of carbohydrates as the hare in this story, bounding rambunctiously about the bloodstream, spiking, crashing, and getting stored away, causing energy to crash. Fat, the tortoise in this story, moves into the bloodstream slowly, providing steady, sustainable energy. Both fat and carbohydrates are forms of fuel, but only carbohydrates cause a spike followed by a crash.

Slow and steady wins the race

Fat provides us with more sustainable energy compared to carbohydrates. Because of this, the brain prefers fat to carbohydrates as its optimal fuel, especially when we are eating at a deficit.

The fat you want to lose is not the fat in food!

Are you concerned that you're trying to lose fat and I'm encouraging you to eat fat? Does it seem contradictory? It's not. The fat (or calories) in your fat cells is harmful. The fat in food can be helpful for stabilizing blood sugar and calming your brain while you lose weight.

They are not the same thing — at all.

The fat in food is a source of useable fuel for both the brain and the body, similar to carbohydrates. The difference is that fat doesn't spike blood sugar and hence does not trigger insulin. It's always burned as fuel as long as we're not overeating. Conversely, carbohydrates continually run the risk of spiking blood sugar and being stored in fat cells, regardless of how many calories we're consuming.

Fat is our friend

Weight loss is a tough task, let's be honest. It requires discipline and determination. Fat helps make the grind a bit easier. In addition to being steady, supportive, and sustaining, fat protects the brain, nervous system, and cell membranes. It also helps balance our mental state and moods. Finally, fat keeps cortisol at bay so that when Tinkerbell starts whispering her sweet nothings into our ear, we can tune in to Jiminy Cricket's voice of reason.

4. Don't jack blood sugar at breakfast

Stabilizing blood sugar begins at breakfast.

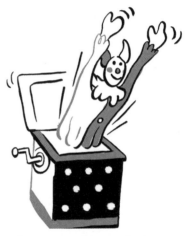

When we wake up in the morning, not having eaten for many hours, we can be fairly certain that our blood sugar is dipping pretty low.

We must tiptoe cautiously, and gently rouse our blood sugar levels and our brain back to a balanced state. We don't want to wind them up like a Jack-in-the-Box. Low blood sugar is most sensitive to the impacts of a high carbohydrate meal. Eating a big bowl of cereal first thing in the morning is asking for trouble.

Take a walk down the cereal aisle of your grocery store and look at the nutrition labels. Pick up a box of the healthy, high-fibre blend marketed to adults. Then look at the cereal made especially for children's palates. Compare them. You'll be shocked at how similar they are beneath the packaging.

The primary ingredient in cereal is glucose. The same goes for bread and granola. Sweetened or not, all grains are full of glucose. All whole or refined grains — gluten-free or gluten-laden — are loaded with glucose. Vanilla and fruit yogurts are spiked with sugar. Don't be misled by the label.

Remember: all carbohydrates break down into sugar.

Banishing beloved breakfast beliefs.

We may argue that we ate these same foods as kids, and that our parents and grandparents had toast and jam their entire lives, and they didn't get fat. Or maybe they did. It doesn't matter. These days we eat more abundantly and gluttonously than ever before. For most people, blood sugar is completely out of whack, the brain is irate, and insulin is rampant.

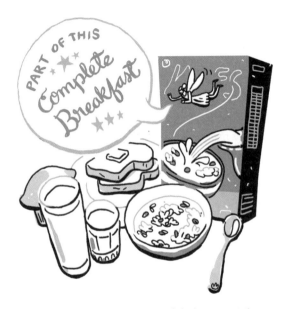

While we're looking at nutrition labels, we might as well read the side of a carton of milk. A cup of 2% milk has 12 grams of sugar, from lactose or glucose added in its place. That's not a *lot*, but it adds to that ever-growing tally. Many of us would never guess we'd been eating so much sugar at breakfast. Glucose on top of glucose, our so-called healthy breakfast is as sweet as a dipped donut.

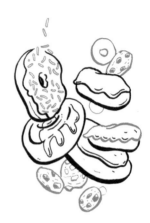

Best bets for breakfast include a choice of eggs, greens, olive oil, protein powder, fruit, nuts and seeds, cottage cheese, and unsweetened Greek yogurt.

5. Eat Snacks to Keep Steady

If we've had the right fuel for breakfast, we should cruise contentedly through the morning, towards lunch, with a consistent level of energy, a clear mind, and a steady mood — all signs that we are burning food as fuel rather than storing it as fat. We may not even feel hungry. These are the signs to look for.

Don't wait for hunger!

The secret to maintaining stable blood sugar is to eat every few hours, before we feel hungry. Once hunger has struck, our blood sugar has already taken a nosedive. Cortisol will be released and it will cause cravings for sugar. Waiting to feel hungry before snacking only makes it more difficult to avoid dense carbohydrates.

Snacks are like training wheels. Their purpose is to keep us steady and to prevent the crash. During any period of weight loss, in particular, eating protein and fat prevents blood sugar drops and minimizes cravings; it allows calories to be released from fat stores to be burned for energy.

A mid-morning snack means we'll make it to lunch in a rational, reasonable state of mind — and it's easier to make wise lunch choices if blood sugar hasn't hit rock bottom when the bell rings.

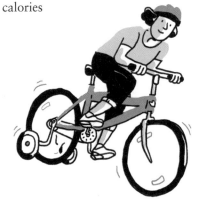

Keepers of the peace

Another way to think of snacks is as peacekeepers. They keep our brain feeling safe and secure — at ease, free of stress and worry. It's under these circumstances only that it will release the fuel stored in our fat cells so we can burn it for the energy we need.

Both high and low blood sugar levels disrupt our mental peace, setting off the brain's panic alarm, sending insulin and cortisol racing out to protect the body. Snacks help keep blood sugar levels steady — and the brain, too, as a result.

In order to begin to minimize calories and empty out the stockroom, the brain has to be relaxed — alert and focused, yes — but calm. This is the purpose of snacks.

What to eat for snacks?

Nuts and seeds make the best snacks. A quarter cup of either is roughly 150 to 180 calories, depending on the variety. A balanced food, containing protein, fat, and carbohydrate, they're convenient, compact, portable, and they keep blood sugar in check for hours, which in turn keeps the insulin-cortisol power struggle at bay. If you're fortunate enough not to be allergic to them and you don't live or work in an environment where they're not permitted, eat them midway between meals.

Do you ever get a surprise visit around four p.m. from the Cookie Monster? He comes to visit many of us at that same time. It's usually the result of a hefty glucose lunch and a crash, or

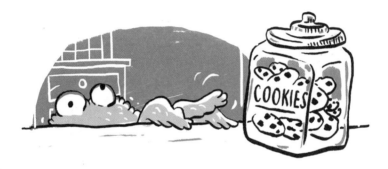

skipping that afternoon snack. Cookie Monster knows our weakness for chocolate chip cookies is greatest when blood sugar is on the floor.

6. Don't let wine and other alcohol throw you off balance.

And, finally, be careful with wine, beer, and alcohol. The same way that alcohol will send you teetering off balance, the sugar in these drinks will quickly throw blood sugar out of whack. A single glass of wine, a beer, or a cocktail can easily add 20 grams of sugar to the meal tally.

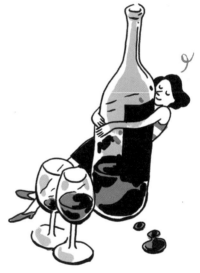

If we're going to indulge in a glass of wine at a meal, then it is especially critical that all other carbohydrates come from green and fibrous vegetables that are nutrient-rich and low in glucose.

It always comes back to the brain.

The brain has the last word about whether we burn food as fuel or store it in fat cells. In order to lose weight we must burn all of the food we're eating as well as the calories stored in fat. When we eat in a way that keeps blood sugar levels steady, the brain is content, and we can begin to empty out the stockroom.

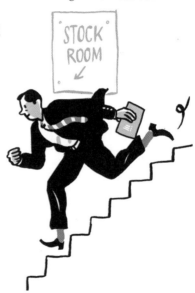

MINIMIZE: THE SECOND PRINCIPLE

Empty Out the Stockroom

This is Bill. He is a shop owner who's been running a successful business for many years. Whatever he orders, he sells — inventory in, inventory out. Nothing accumulates in the stockroom. Then, for no apparent reason, business takes a turn. Sales begin to slow down, yet Bill keeps ordering the same quantity of merchandise. The inventory starts to pile up. His business begins to suffer.

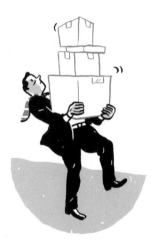

The body is our business. Our fat cells are our stockroom.

In the same way that Bill's business suffers when inventory piles up in his stockroom, our body suffers when calories pile up in our fat cells. When we're stashing food away, we aren't sellingit. If this continues, the bodyswells in size and becomes sluggish. In time, vital processes stop functioning as they should.

To lose weight we must minimize the calories we are consuming so as to deplete the calories we are storing.

Calories are inventory

Think of eating food as ordering inventory. When we burn the calories in food to produce energy, we're selling inventory. When inventory piles up in fat cells, we get fat. To lose weight, we have to get rid of this extra inventory.

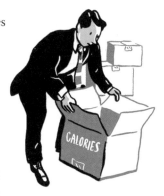

We can only empty fat cells by ordering less inventory — consuming fewer calories — for an ongoing period of time. While the minimizing of calories must be substantial, it must be done strategically so that the brain is continually willing to dip into fat cells for the calories it needs.

It's resourceful to use what we already have in stock, especially when it comes to the body. Getting rid of excess calories is not only sensible, it's vital. An accumulation of fuel in our fat cells is harmful.

Minimizing means dieting

Emptying the stockroom means eating less. We won't lose weight by eating the same amount of calories we are eating now, no matter how healthy they are. That is the bad news. The good news is we don't have to be on a deficit forever. Just long enough to lose the weight.

It comes down to one undeniable truth. If we're eating the same number of calories as we always have, there is no need for more fuel.

However, when we cut back on the calories we eat while maintaining stable blood sugar levels, we will dip into fat cells for the remaining fuel we need. When we keep dipping in, day after day, week after week, we lose weight.

Minimizing is a committed depletion period that depends on ongoing caloric subtraction. We must be eating at a continual deficit, with determination and conviction. The objective is simple; to under-eat, strategically and carefully, so that the calories in our fat cells are liberated into the bloodstream and burned as fuel for our energy demands.

Minimizing means deficit

Minimizing is often confused with healthy eating. While it can and should be executed in a healthy way, minimizing always means eating at a deficit for an extended period of time.

Both stabilizing and minimizing involve blood sugar and the brain, but minimizing is strictly about cutting back on calories in order to empty inventory from fat cells.

The math has to work

We lose weight through a process of ongoing subtraction. When we continually take away from the calorie reserve in fat cells, without adding it back the next day, we lose weight.

If we burn 2,000 calories a day and eat 1,500, that's 500 calories fewer than what we need. The missing 500 calories can then be taken from our fat cells, assuming that blood sugar levels are steady. If we do this every day, while staying under the brain's panic radar, in a week we can lose a pound.

If we take 500 calories out of fat cells every day by eating at a 500 calorie deficit, we'll have no trouble losing 20 pounds in five months. When we add exercise into the mix, that deficit can be doubled, hastening weight loss.

The subtraction is simple. The tough part is keeping at it. The minimizing must happen day after day, for weeks or months, depending on how much weight we may need to lose. The more conviction we have, the sooner the weight will come off.

If we're subtracting calories every day for an extended time, we'll easily lose weight. On the other hand, if we subtract calories one day and then add them back the next, we aren't minimizing. It still equalizes, like an irresistible force meeting up with an immovable object. That is inertia.

If we're losing a pound a week for over a month we can be pretty sure we've mastered strategic subtraction. And it isn't necessary to obsess about counting all the calories we eat. If we aren't losing weight, we can assume that we aren't minimizing correctly or enough. We must minimize and stabilize further. The body will figure out the rest.

As we get rid of the calories stored in fat cells, there will no longer be a need for all that space. Think of it like downsizing from a mansion to a condo. When you get rid of all that dense, bulky furniture, a smaller space will do. So, the body shrinks its storage space, becomes more compact. This is why burning stored calories makes us physically smaller.

While we may want to empty our fat cells of stored calories for both weight and health reasons, the brain, in its protective nature, isn't so eager to relinquish its hoardings. It has worked very hard, with the help of insulin, to stash away these calories; it's not looking to give them up. So, while we're minimizing food intake, we'd better stay below the brain's panic alarm.

Staying below the brain's panic alarm

Both high and low blood sugar, along with excessive under-eating, will cause the brain to hold tighter to its hoardings. The same factors that cause weight gain also inhibit the loss of it. All weight

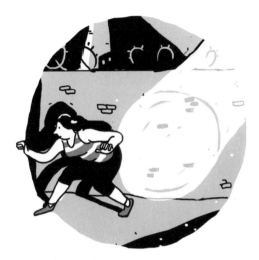

loss efforts will collapse if we don't tend to the brain at all times.

If we start skipping meals, avoiding protein and scrimping on fat, the brain will clue in to the fact that we're trying to steal from its savings while also depriving it of essential nutrition. Not a wise move. If, on the other hand, we're under-eating in a way that stabilizes, satisfies, and sustains the brain, then it will relax and release some of the calories it has been hoarding in fat cells.

We can't cut calories recklessly or haphazardly. The first principle of stabilizing can never be abandoned: minimizing must be done on a stable foundation of balanced blood sugar. The subtraction must be strategically executed.

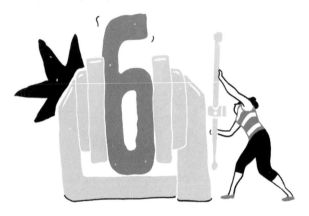

There are six strategies for minimizing:

1. Pack only essential calories
2. Shrink your lunch
3. Stretch calories

4. Fill up on greens
5. Eat snacks to keep the minimizing going
6. Live like a minimalist

1. Pack Only the Essentials

On this weight loss journey, we have to travel light, eatingonly essential foods, leaving out the rest. We want maximum nutrition for minimal calories. Protein, fat, and vegetables are our passport, compass, and a

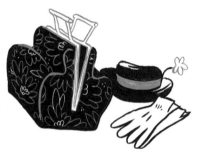

fresh change of clothes. We want to eat only the most nutrient-dense foods, so that any missing fuel will come from fat cells.

The only way to eat well, while on a deficit, is to leave out those foods that have the greatest density of sugar and calories and the least amount of nutrition. If we want to access the fuel in our fat cells, then we may have to relinquish a few of our favourite foods.

While many foods may be wholesome and natural, continuing to eat them won't create the deficit we need for weight loss. Dense carbohydrates are a form of useable fuel, but they are also full of calories and sugar. Don't fret, there will be bread again. For now, stay to the course until the finish line. This is the race the hare doesn't win.

2. Shrink Your Lunch

While bread has become a staple lunch box item, we'll survive without it. Lunch is best kept small and to the essentials. There are a few reasons for this. Many of us spend much of the day sitting. (If you're a bike courier or mail carrier, this doesn't apply to you, though you may find a hefty lunch doesn't serve you well) either.

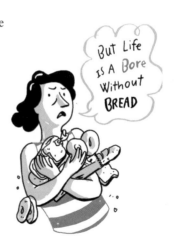

No matter how hard we may be thinking at work, sitting doesn't demand many calories in comparison to moving. A big lunch will only spike blood sugar and insulin, ending up in fat cells — which doesn't do much good for the brain or weight loss. Remember, we're trying to empty our stockroom, not fill it up.

Leave the brain alone while it's trying to think

In order to keep the brain content while relinquishing calorie hoardings, we have to tiptoe under its panic radar. Hitting the food court for a hearty sandwich or a 700-calorie salad is not the way to do this. Regardless of how wholesome it is, a big meal will inevitably lead to an insulin spike, a storage of calories, a cortisol rush, and a blood sugar crash.

Have you ever wondered why you can't keep your eyes open come two p.m.? It's not likely that you didn't eat enough. It's likely that you ate too much, or too many carbohydrates. Remember the insulin sugar defence team, racing though the bloodstream, rounding up all that glucose fuel and storing it in fat cells? That's exactly what has happened when we need a nap after lunch.

Have a light lunch — have a liquid lunch

A shake, a soup, or a small salad is more than sufficient for the working brain. Think of lunch as a snack, only slightly more substantial. Another fuel top-up to keep blood sugar and energy levels steady. The last thing we want at lunch is to dump inventory back into the stockroom we're trying to empty.

Midday is as good a time as any for a mental break and physical movement. Resist the urge to hit the food court. Go for a walk instead. A brisk midday walk is a better alternative than eating excess, unnecessary calories.

Once the weight is off, we can revert to slightly larger lunches if we so desire; but by then, we'll likely be enjoying the mental benefits of eating less in the middle of the day. We'll be alert at two p.m., not sleepy.

3. Stretch calories.

A smaller amount of food stretched over a longer period of time results in fewer calories consumed over the course of the day. The more carefully and consistently we stretch calories — without triggering low blood sugar or hunger — the more continuous weight loss will be.

Think of the process like an elastic band. An elastic band can easily extend an inch, but if we continue to stretch it, it may extend three or four inches. It depends on how careful we are about it — and knowing when we're taking it too far.

By stretching calories, we flatten out the spikes and dips in our blood sugar. Eating vegetables makes it easy. It doesn't work so well with grains.

Have you ever made zucchini noodles?

By substituting sautéed zucchini strips for pasta, we can stretch a high calorie meal into two smaller meals and still feel satisfied while ensuring that we're maintaining stable blood sugar levels.

Zucchini can be a fine substitute for pasta. Sliced in thin strips, it makes a perfect base for Bolognese or any tomato-based or lighter sauce. It holds its shape and adds texture to a dish, yet contributes few calories to the meal. An entire zucchini has fewer calories than a single forkful of pasta.

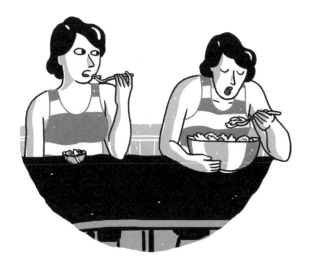

Part of what we enjoy — and what we often miss while we're trying to lose weight — is the physical action of eating and the social satisfaction that comes with sharing food. We like to talk over a meal, laugh, and swirl. We can enjoy all of this, if we know which foods allow us to stretch calories across a meal.

4. Fill up on greens

We can fill up on greens with reckless abandon, in glorious abundance, and still be minimizing calories. We can eat bowls full and still not have consumed many calories. Our belly will be satisfied long before we've eaten too many.

Kale, collards, broccoli, arugula, spinach, rapini, broccolini, Swiss chard, beet greens, dandelion, watercress, parsley, and lettuces … the list goes on and on. The magic of greens lies in the fact that they're so densely packed with fibre and water, along with minerals, vitamins, and antioxidants, that there's no room for glucose and calories. We can eat greens to our heart's content and still not have eaten an excess of calories.

Not all vegetables are created equal

Roots and tubers are very different from greens due to their caloric and carbohydrate density. They are more like grains. A few bites of potato is equivalent to a few forkfuls of pasta, and may spike blood sugar in the same way. Better to stick to the greens.

*Half a cup of cooked sweet potato equals
twelve cups of raw spinach or arugula*

All vegetables are good, but in order to burn the calories sitting in fat cells, the subtraction has to be continuous. During this subtraction stage, when choosing which carbohydrates to eat, the secret is this: maximum nutrition for minimal calories.

Just because we're abstaining from certain foods right now doesn't mean we'll never eat them again. There will be plenty of time later to enjoy them. For now, however, we have to let the calorie deficit do its work.

Part of the strategy with weight loss involves cutting back on any fuel the brain and body won't miss. This is the only sure way to empty out the stockroom while still enjoying cooking and eating, and getting an adequate dose of daily nutrition.

Why not take the path of least resistance?

5. Eat Snacks to Keep the Minimizing Going

Why do endurance athletes take in snacks during a race? Is it to cover all the calories they're burning? No. They'd have to be eating constantly, which would detract from their performance — since blood would be diverted away from muscle to digest food. The purpose of these snacks is to keep their brain calm, blood sugar levels stable, and to provide a small amount of 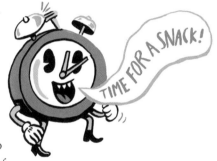 fuel, while fat cells and muscle glycogen offer up the rest.

Our snacks have a similar purpose. Their aim is to keep the brain content, while providing only partially the calories we need. These small fuel inputs maintain steady blood sugar, so the brain allows us to take additional calories from our fat cells.

And, no, we won't be sucking back energy gels like the guys in the Tour de France. If we were running a four-hour race, a hit of glucose might be useful, but since most of us spend the day sitting down, our snacks will not include simple sugars.

Remember; the unwavering foundation for weight loss is stable blood sugar levels. No matter how minimal our calorie intake may be, if snacks are spiking blood sugar and insulin, we will have a tougher time shedding the weight.

6. Think Like a Minimalist.

Instead of thinking of how unfortunate it is that we can't eat as much as we'd like to, try looking at it from a different perspective. It is as wasteful to buy and bring home food that we don't need as it is to eat it and see it go to waste in our fat cells.

Why do we fill our cupboards and pack our fridges? What would happen if we stopped stocking our kitchens full of all the foods that we may indeed want but don't need?

The more food we buy, the more food we feel compelled to eat, and the harder it is to affect positive change concerning our weight and health. Not to mention that the more food we buy the more waste we produce. The carbon footprint of food production, packaging, and transportation is staggering.

In a weight loss sense, minimizing means fewer calories sitting in our fat cells. In a global sense it means consuming and wasting less food. When we minimize calories from food in order to subtract from calories in fat cells, we will be buying less food. This may seem like a small feat, but if millions of us did this, the universal impact would be far greater than a few pounds lost.

Minimize manipulation

Alongside the increase in average body size in North America, there has been a parallel and paradoxical increase in our awareness and understanding of the addictive tendencies of the brain and our knowledge of the food industry's motivations. How can this be? We would think that having a deeper understanding of the fragile brain and the body's reactions to certain foods (sugar) would make us want to protect them from eating habits that trigger addictive and harmful responses. Instead, the food industry uses food as a handy device to manipulate the brain's conflicting desires. More now than at any time in recorded history, food is being marketed and consumed for entertainment and short-lived enjoyment.

How Do We Know We're Minimizing Correctly?

When we are executing the subtraction successfully we'll know. The results will be obvious. If we keep below the panic radar while emptying the stockroom, we'll experience mental clarity and weight loss, simultaneously. When the minimizing is done right, the brain is content, it functions better and it will give up its hoardings. The deficit stage will eventually come to an end, but it takes time. If the pounds fall away too quickly, there's reason to be concerned. Safely depleting our fat cells of the unnecessary calories we've collected requires patience and persistence.

The weight will come off. The science and the math work. We can tweak things, as long as we steer clear of the brain's insulin-cortisol radar. If we're losing weight, feeling clear-headed and free of cravings, we're on the right track.

Back to the analogy of Bob and his store: the more we sell and the less we order, the more quickly we will empty our stockroom. If we eat 2,000 calories a day and we burn 2,000 calories a day, then no matter how healthily we're eating, we won't lose weight. Healthy eating alone does not lead to weight loss. We only empty fat cells when we aren't eating enough food. It's the difference between what our body burns in a day and what we are consuming that causes us to lose weight.

However stable our blood sugar may be and however many greens we may be eating, we won't shed a pound if we're eating as much as our body burns in a day.

When we hit inertia

When we hit inertia, which we will, we'll have to adjust, and likely minimize further. But even still, focusing on food alone won't be sufficient. All the minimizing and stabilizing in the world won't take off the weight long-term without the help of exercise, the third principle.

Exercise overcomes inertia

Without exercise, weight loss will eventually come to a screeching halt. It is the dynamic force that pulls weight loss along. More importantly, exercise prevents the weight from returning after we've finished the minimizing stage.

EXERCISE:
THE THIRD
PRINCIPLE

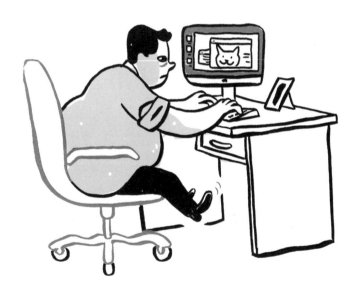

We live in bodies that are lined with muscles evolved for movement and work — and a lot of it. These muscles are connected to bones and joints, to a cardiovascular and nervous system, all connected by wiring to the brain. And yet, most of us sit all day and then we lie down all night.

We tend to lead sedentary lives, which is not healthy regardless of our weight. Aside from eating too much food — and too many of the wrong kinds of foods — the main reason we gain unnecessary weight in the first place is because we spend much of our lives sitting.

Exercise powers weight loss

Exercise can be considered the magic button that powers the first two principles. Movement and muscle activate the body's calorie-burning potential.

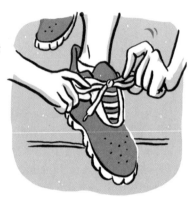

In time — and only once the weight is off — dense muscle will allow us to eat more calories without gaining all the weight back — within reason. But during weight-loss, rewarding hard workouts with more food will only send us chasing our tails. Exercise can never override the effects of over-eating.

The Body Is Structured for Movement

A big part of the solution to our weight woes lies in realigning our lives with the natural ways and workings of the body.

The structure of the body, from the head down to the heel, is ideal for agile, spring-like movement. We have a powerful gluteus maximus that didn't evolve to fill a pair of jeans or a comfortable couch. Its job is to stabilize and propel us forward. We sit on it all day long, but this is not its actual purpose.

Movement and muscle

Activity alone can never override imbalanced blood sugar or over-eating. But when exercise is combined with the first two principles, miracles happen. Inertia is surpassed. Both cardiovascular and strength training increase our vigour and vitality, pulling weight loss along.

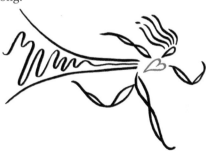

By building strong muscle, we boost the body's metabolism, so that once we lose the weight, it won't climb back on again. Muscle is like a storage tank for extra fuel — a better one than fat cells. When we have dense muscle, any extra calories we eat will be compacted into muscle rather than going back to fat cells.

Three reasons why exercise is essential to weight loss:

1. Moving burns more calories than sitting, lying down, or sleeping. No matter how much we ponder, problem solve, or make profound discoveries, thinking never burns more calories than moving. Moving also stimulates the nervous system, and increases our body's ability to produce energy. When we combine increased activity with fewer calories, weight loss is easier.

2. Active muscle is under constant construction. After a workout, the body uses calories to build and repair muscle, making it stronger and more resilient. When we lift, push, or pull against a force, muscles adapt to the work we've demanded of them by tearing during a workout and then repairing afterwards. This burns a lot of calories.

3. Muscle boosts metabolism and prevents fat cells from filling up again. It helps if we think of it as expensive real estate. The property taxes and maintenance fees for muscle tissue are much higher than for fat cells. It takes hundreds more calories to maintain muscle than it does to maintain fat. When our metabolism is higher, we can eat more food without getting fat. Strength training also prevents the natural muscle atrophy that comes with age, so we don't have to eat less and less, with each passing year.

There are two forms of exercise:

1. *Daily cardiovascular activity*
    Aerobic exercise at a lower intensity, such as walking, skipping, hiking, jogging, or cycling burns far more calories than sitting down, and is essential for emptying out the stockroom. Unless you're an avid athlete, walking is the most important activity.

2. *Strength training*
    Anaerobic exercise also burns calories, both during and after the activity; first we overload and tear, and then we repair and

rebuild the muscles we've just worked. The more muscle we have on our frame, the faster our metabolism will be. With time and effort, our body will burn more calories every day, even while we're sitting around doing nothing. This is the greatest perk muscle provides.

There are six strategies for exercise:

1. Be wary of high intensity cardio
2. Walk
3. Build muscle
4. Don't eat away your exercise
5. Bite off what you can chew
6. Be committed

1. Be Wary of High Intensity Cardio

It's easy to chase our tails when it comes to exercise and weight loss, and many forms of exercise can do this. The primary culprit is activity that's too intense, especially when combined with a calorie deficit. Be careful.

While exercise is critical to both well-being and weight loss, it's also a form of physical stress. Be careful of cortisol. High-intensity cardiovascular exercise will add extra stress on top of life's everyday stresses. This can quickly send us back down the rabbit hole of cortisol release, sugar cravings, carbohydrate consumption leading to high blood sugar, followed by insulin release, low blood sugar, cortisol, and further cravings.

When activity sends our heart rate soaring, the brain demands sugar as it is the quickest fuel for this type of activity. This isn't what we necessarily want. What we want to be using the fuel that is sitting in our fat cells. Slow the cardio, steady the heart.

If you're already an athlete, then you may be fine with higher intensity activity — even while on a calorie deficit — since your body has already learned how to access fuel from fat cells. But if you aren't an athlete, less intense, longer duration cardiovascular exercise will likely work better for weight loss, so you can burn the fuel in fat cells without being nagged by constant carbohydrate cravings.

2. Walk

You may be wondering why — with the plethora of hard-core exercise regimes — I would be recommending something as simple, as enjoyable as walking.

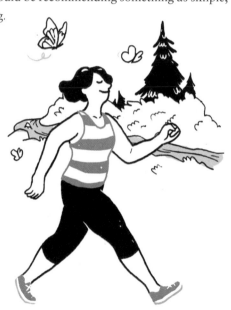

While we're on a calorie deficit, the brain is especially sensitive to the additional calorie demands of exercise. Because walking is done at a lower, sustained heart rate, it manages to slip under the brain's radar, while emptying out the stockroom.

Remember the first principle,

stabilizing blood sugar? Its primary intention is to keep the brain at peace, to allow for minimizing without sending it into a panic. The brain must also be content with how we are exercising, which can be a challenging

endeavour when we're already eating at a deficit. Exercise, when added to minimizing, is asking the brain to release more of the stored fuel.

During the minimizing stage, we must be cognitive of the efforts we are demanding from our body and our brain. If we start jacking up our heart rate, we're playing with fire. Be careful! Remember that the calories in our fat cells are the brain's precious stockroom of hoarded fuel. We must tiptoe cautiously as we take from its prized stash.

Walking keeps the peace

When we exercise in a way that keeps cortisol at bay, we can take more fuel from the stockroom while not messing around with our blood sugar and our brain.

If you've been running for a few years, then your cardiovascular fitness is likely advanced enough that you will gradually switch from burning carbohydrates as your primary fuel for activity to burning the fuel stored in fat cells instead, without feeling wonky or craving sugar afterwards. If this is the case, then by all means, continue to do what you've been doing.

But if you don't like running, if it elevates your stress levels, or if you always crave carbohydrates for hours after, then running may not your ideal exercise choice while minimizing your calorie intake. The same applies if you've been going to spinning classes committedly for months, sweating out your soul, and still haven't taken off a pound. It's time to start walking.

Here's the thing. If you've been embarking on ambitious workouts at a high intensity and you haven't lost any weight — maybe you've even gained weight — then it's time to try something new.

Walk one hour every day and the weight will come off

Why I walk

If you're getting the sense that I am partial to walking, you're right. As a teenager, I started travelling about the city on foot. Born to parents who had neither car nor licence, I got around by walking or by taking public transit, more often the former due to impatience with waiting for buses. I would walk to the next stop, then the next, and then just kept on going, forgetting to look back for the bus until it drove past.

By the start of high school, walking had slipped into my everyday routine. I'd sneak out of school at lunchtime to wander the downtown for an hour, and then walk much of the way home after class, with reluctantly abiding friends.

Back then, I never thought of walking as having anything to do with physical fitness or mental well-being. It was just something I did because I liked being outside and enjoyed the freedom of wandering. By the time I was in my early twenties, walking an hour a day became a ritual. Especially after leaving home, when everything was suddenly new and unfamiliar, walking maintained a sense of normality in my life.

It also became a way to keep my mind at ease. This was a gradual and profound discovery that became most evident on the days when I didn't walk. Something felt amiss, although I couldn't pinpoint exactly why. Skipping that daily venture on foot left me with a sense of unsettledness.

It wasn't until many years later, and with further education, that I came to understand the connection between walking, well-being (physical and mental), and weight loss. Walking is one of the simplest of activities and yet it works wonders.

Exercise is often thought best when it is a vigorous endeavour — harder, faster, more! We're encouraged to jack our heart rates up, higher and higher still. For training purposes, this is fine and good, but it doesn't necessarily pair well with weight loss.

Harder and faster are not always the right courses of action. Exercising at moderate intensity with a sustained heart rate is not insignificant, especially when done regularly. Quite the opposite, in fact; it is very significant to our well-being. Most of us have more than enough stress in our lives already, so a form of activity that can lower stress levels rather than raise them is exactly what we need.

In combination with stable blood sugar and caloric subtraction, walking is a sure way to hasten the emptying of fuel from fat cells. If we're consistent with the first two principles and then start walking an hour every day, the results will be dramatic.

A quick thirty-minute walk at lunchtime can burn up to two hundred calories. The amount depends on the pace or level of exertion and, of course, the person's size and weight. Add another thirty minutes and the real magic happens. Walking an hour a day for a year can burn thirty pounds of calories.

If walking isn't something you enjoy, find another activity you do like — and one that won't cause you to crave sugar. The benefit of walking is that you can do it every day. The body, the brain, and weight loss all work best with regular movement.

Two reasons walking works for weight loss:

1. It hastens the subtraction of calories from fat cells
2. It does this without alarming the brain

While minimizing calorie intake, exercise must be done subtly and strategically. No matter how many calories we may think we're burning, the brain has the final word.

Let's say we've been walking for a full year, have listened to ninety audio books, have learned a new language, and have lost thirty pounds. That's an astonishing feat. We've managed to burn thousands of stored calories, all the while keeping our brain content. Good work!

Once the weight is off, we may feel confident that we can now start eating baskets of bread again and adding all those grains back into our meals. Better rethink that idea. Thanks to all the cardio, stabilizing, and minimizing, we may indeed have emptied fat cells of extra inventory, but it's too easy to dump it all right back in again, especially since the body doesn't require as much food now.

A smaller body needs less fuel

Weight loss makes our body smaller, which means we need less food. It doesn't seem fair to lose all that weight — a noble undertaking — only to be destined to a life of having to eat fewer calories than we ate while dieting. This is the not-so-sad reality that befalls every person, post-diet, who presumes that, after losing weight, they can safely revert back to their old ways of eating. But it doesn't work that way. Being smaller means we need less food to fuel us, unless we equip ourselves with muscle.

3. Build muscle

Muscle makes and keeps us lean. Since our concern here is weight loss, let's look at the reasons why muscle is vital to losing weight, keeping it off, and improving overall health.

Muscle is a compact fuel tank for storing extra calories. Fat cells also store calories but in an unhealthy, flabby way.

Muscle is lean, useful, and densely packed. By building muscle we build a better tank than fat cells for storing extra fuel.

Muscle is able to condense extra calories into a small space where they are both useful and easy to access.

Muscle is the most active tissue in the body, thanks to a plethora of mitochondria — the part of the cell where calories are converted into energy.

Muscle has the capacity to store extra calories that we have no immediate use for in a small, safe, compact space, known as glycogen. When we need more energy, we can easily access the fuel stored in muscle glycogen and burn it for energy. Without a dense supply of active muscle lining our frame, many of the calories we consume will get socked away in fat cells — where the words small, safe, and compact do not apply.

Use it, or lose it

As we age, we lose muscle. Without regular strength training, it is an unavoidable fate for all of us. Aside from an increased risk of falling and fractures, the progressive atrophy of muscle drags our metabolism down. This makes weight loss nearly impossible and weight gain inevitable. We don't want to lose our muscle. We want to build more of it.

Build muscle, boost metabolism

With muscle lining our frame, not only are we firmer and leaner, it becomes much harder to fill fat cells back up again. If we're working muscle against resistance on a regular basis, we're burning hundreds or thousands of calories, rather than storing them.

The harder we train, the more energy we need and thus the more calories we burn. This doesn't mean we should start eating more. Don't jump ahead! For now, keep minimizing. Once the weight has been lost, then we can rest assured that we'll be able to eat a bit more food without gaining all that weight back again — a sign that our metabolism has kicked into a higher gear.

By building muscle, we make our body into a powerful food processor, so that after we've diligently lost the weight, we don't pack it back on again a year or two later.

When we invest in building muscle, we increase our metabolism. The stronger we become, the greater our capacity for processing food into energy, regardless of size. Muscle is a powerful fuel processor compared to a crappy blender.

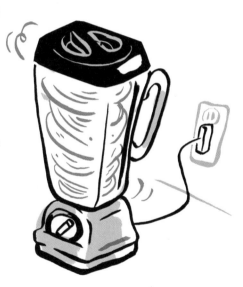

Muscle keeps our metabolic engine firing on all

cylinders. We want a strong metabolism, not one that's slow and sluggish and quick to store food in fat. While walking will tiptoe under the brain's radar, allowing us to burn stored fuel, it is not enough to keep the weight off. To prevent the weight from piling back on again after the diet is done, muscle is the answer.

Building muscle is the surest and only way to avoid the ultimate future of having to eat less and less food. With dense muscle and stable blood sugar levels we will lose the weight and not gain it all back again. Skinny is not the same as lean. Lean means muscle. Muscle means you can eat more.

Muscle Increases Vitality

Aside from the obvious physical differences between fat and muscle, the more significant but unknown difference between the two is that fat perpetuates the dangerous domino effect, while muscle stops the dominoes from falling.

Fuel in Muscle Is Useful, Not Harmful

By building muscle, we build a much safer fuel tank than fat cells. In fact, muscle can undo some of the damage that has already been set in motion by a high carbohydrate diet, beginning with emptying fat cells of stored calories and burning them as fuel.

Storing calories in muscle does not perpetuate high cortisol levels, inflammation, or any of the other ricochet reactions that arise from excess calories being stored in fat cells. During weight loss, as we eat less food and build more muscle, calories are continually diverted away from fat towards muscle. Picture all that stored fuel exiting fat cells and heading over to thriving muscle where work is being done to burn even more excess calories.

There's a catch: you can't build muscle by pushing a button

We don't get stronger muscle by paying for a gym membership, or hanging out in gym clothes, socializing and reading the newspaper. Nor do we increase strength by lifting the same weight we've been lifting for five years. Dumbbells that serve as doorstops also don't transfer their potential usefulness onto our physical frames.

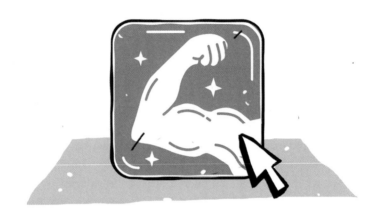

Working against resistance builds muscle

Also known as overload, this is what builds strength. It's hard work. In order to bring about the desired changes in metabolism and body composition, ongoing adaptation must occur within our muscle tissue. The physiological transformations only happen when we exert great force against much resistance. In other words, lifting, moving, pulling or pushing a heavy weight is what brings about change.

Building and maintaining a lean body requires physical labour and mental rigour. You may or may not find pleasure in strength training, initially — it depends on whether you enjoy a physical challenge. In time, however, you'll come to enjoy the aftermath and perhaps the work itself. But don't expect it to be easy. Building muscle is arduous.

How Strength Training Works

During a proper strength-training workout, we should be tearing muscle fibre. This might sound painful, but it's one of the most generous gifts we can offer up to our body and our brain. After the workout, for the next day or two, muscle undergoes a period of repair, during which time the body uses calories to build more resilient and dense muscle fibres. Strength training also sharpens the brain and nervous system.

As we increase the workload, muscle gets stronger and more capable of handling more challenging workouts. The entire body grows more resilient to obesity, illness, and injury, and life's every-day physical and mental demands.

We burn calories both during and after strength training workouts. If we're simultaneously minimizing the calories we're consuming from food — all the while keeping the brain at peace with stable blood sugar — we'll continually dip into fat cells for more fuel.

Fat does not turn into muscle

Contrary to what you may think, fat does not turn into muscle, but rather fat cells liberate stored calories to be used as fuel by the body to perform the work being done by muscles, as well as for their repair and maintenance in between workouts. In other words, fat cells are depleted while muscle is created.

The greater the overload, the more calories will be depleted from fat cells, with increased frequency. With ongoing strength training — in combination with stabilizing and minimizing — the fuel in fat cells will continue to decrease as lean body composition increases.

Think of active muscle as a thriving business that employs calories as fuel to do its work. With a heavy workload, muscle needs more workers to get the job done. So it heads over to fat cell factories to recruit fuel workers that are lazing around. The more work muscle has on the go, the greater its need for calories to fill all the job positions.

Muscle takes idle fuel from fat cells and puts it to work

During the minimizing stage, with blood sugar steady and subtraction continuous, the muscle factory will frequently turn to the fat cell factory for more fuel. Eventually, fat cell factories close up shop as calories leave for more energizing endeavours.

With continued hard work, muscle will thrive, and fat cells will shrivel up. At a certain point, an amazing thing happens. We can eat a bit more food without fat cells filling back up again.

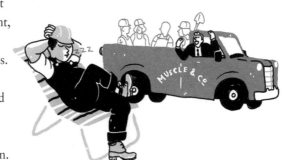

Boring? Better than Being Overweight and Lethargic

You may think that strength training is a bore. That's fair. You may not find it as stimulating as watching television or staring at your phone, but it has a far more positive impact on your nervous system and body composition. There are hundreds of hobbies and activities far more enticing than lifting weights, but none are as smart a strategy for preventing fat cells from filling up again.

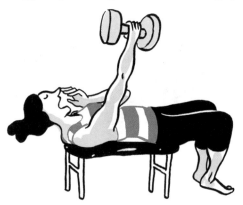

Brushing our teeth can be a drag, but we do it

Most of us spend at least four minutes a day brushing our teeth. (This doesn't include flossing. There's another four minutes.) That's almost an hour a week on our teeth. We do it because we know that, without good dental hygiene, we open our mouths to cavities and bad odours.

Without proper muscle-building habits, we open the door not only to obesity but also to disease.

An hour a week is more than enough time to begin a good strength training routine. Half an hour, twice a week will have a profound impact on our health. Increase that to two hours, and we're sailing towards a leaner, longer life. If it's boring, that's likely a sign that we aren't working hard enough. Hard work is never boring!

Getting started with strength training

1. *Hire a trainer.*

    You don't have to spend thousands of dollars or get a live-in personal trainer, but in order to strength train properly, you'll want to learn how to lift weights correctly, to get the most out of your time, and, most importantly, to prevent injury.

A knowledgeable trainer will teach you the proper form and technique for the most time-efficient, useful exercises for getting stronger.

2. *Focus on the larger muscle groups:* glutes, back, chest, abdominals, and legs.

Why these ones? These are our most powerful muscles, with the greatest capacity for stamina and strength. They burn high amounts of calories during and after each workout and powerfully boost metabolism.

3. *Lift heavy and hard.*

To build muscle, we need overload. The most simple and straightforward program for anyone starting out is to lift a heavy but manageable weight for ten repetitions and repeat this for three sets, all the while maintaining the correct form. A trainer for a few sessions is a wise idea for preventing potential injury.

Remember: the purpose of strength training is to tear and repair muscle. This requires resistance and weight. The workout must be challenging enough that the body has to adapt to it.

4. Don't eat away your exercise.

While we may feel that a hard workout garners reward, even a few gratifying bites can quickly dump all the fuel we just burned back into fat cells. As commendable as our new exercise habits may be, splurging only delays the subtraction. The deficit must be ongoing to keep that weight coming off, otherwise it's a pound off, a pound on, over and over again.

Three slices of pizza is a waste of time more than a deserved reward. The math just doesn't work that way. It takes approximately two minutes to gobble down a few cookies, 1,000 calories of pasta, or a hunk of baguette. Two minutes. That's it. Are those few minutes of self-indulgence worth the hours and days and weeks we are required spend burning off that excess fuel?

Think of the importance of your time
when you eat something that wastes it

It is unfortunate that we have to look at eating this way, but it's also the truth of the matter. The time component is most significant especially if we have a lot of weight to lose. Of course, even with splurges we will lose it, but why not make the journey a little easier and shorter?

Time is scarce for most of us. There is barely enough time in a day to spend it on the people and things that are most important. The least we can do is save ourselves some extra time later by not eating in a way that wastes it. Losing weight takes time. Exercise is essential, in whatever form, and this takes time. It's a vital and wonderful use of time, and one that will leave us feeling more rejuvenated than most other time-sucking things.

But we certainly don't want to be adding to the time that will be needed to take the weight off by consuming an hour or two of exercise in minutes. There are far better ways to spend our time than burning off thousands of calories of stored fuel that took mere minutes to consume.

Ongoing subtraction is what leads to weight loss. When we reward laborious efforts with excess calories, it becomes addition again, the very opposite of what we intended and have been working towards. All those hard-burned calories that we just liberated from our fat cells will pile right back in again with a few ravenous mouthfuls. The math will always override even the greatest of rationalizations. Don't add back what you've just subtracted. Have a salt bath as a reward. Read a good book.

Muscle won't forgive gluttony

After the weight is lost, we can certainly have pizza or pasta from time-to-time without fear of refilling our fat cells, but there is no room for excessive consumption, no matter how much muscle we've built. While building active, dense muscle can allow more leeway with eating, muscle and exercise can never override excess food. You can't out-walk or out-run bad eating habits.

5. Bite Off What You Can Chew

While we may feel highly motivated to get the weight off right now, this momentum won't last forever. It may not last a week if it's too ambitious. Though we may be committed to losing the weight, there are still the same number of hours and obligations in a week. No amount of optimism can alter the unchangeable aspects of busy everyday living.

Be realistic

Before committing to seven days a week at the gym, it's worth contemplating the reality of our lives and how exercise will fit in. How long will an overly ambitious program last before we kick it to the curb? Being realistic, even a tad pessimistic, will save us from disappointment and despair in the course of those first few weeks. An all-consuming, seven-day-a-week gym routine that we soon quit is of no use for getting into shape.

6. Be Committed

We have to commit. Getting stronger and leaner takes work. In time we might even enjoy it. Building muscle takes effort. Walking takes time. Exercise demands persistence and wholehearted dedication. It's a decision that you have to make and remake every day. When we begin weight training, a leap of faith is required if we've never done it before. We may wonder how all of this tear and repair can actually be good for us, when all it seems to do now is make us sore. Perhaps the best way to think of physical activity is like a long-term partnership, because that's what it has to be. If the joy of exercise is gone after a few short days, then the weight loss we're seeking won't ever materialize.

With persistence, the changes will come

We may wonder how we'll find the time or energy for any of this. How can we commit more time when we don't have an extra second to ourselves right now? The time will appear if the results are worthwhile. And they are. Being stronger provides more energy to accomplish more in a day.

Living in line with the body

The thing we tend to forget is that we don't get to decide what the body needs. It has evolved a certain way, and all we can do is learn and understand the workings of it, if we so choose. If the body has become sluggish it's because we're not moving enough and we're eating too much, or incorrectly. When we eat less and move more, the body starts to work right. It's quite simple if we are willing to see how simple it is.

The perks of exercise go beyond the pounds

There is a reason exercise is considered a form of therapy or an alternative to drugs or other highs. Activity stimulates the brain. It is its own reward. Anyone who's highly active will attest to this. As the physical transformations set in, the mental benefits come alongside. Right now we may not believe that this can be possible, but it is.

If we're feeling low and sluggish, it's a daunting task to push ourselves physically. The last thing we feel like doing is exerting strength. But the rewards will appear soon after starting, and they'll be well worth the effort.

GET THE
BRAIN ON
BOARD

Stabilize, minimize, exercise: knowing these three principles is one thing. Living them is another. It is possible, of course, to follow the principles without buying groceries, prepping food, or even turning on the stove. You can, in actuality, eat all your meals in restaurants, or on the run, and still lose weight. It will be more challenging, a great deal more costly, and likely deficient in green vegetables, but it is nonetheless possible.

And then there is the brain to contend with

Get the brain on board. The first thing we want to get in order is our brain. It has to be on board. We need it rooting for us here because how we think precedes how we act. When we know what has to happen and then plan for it, our actions will be clear.

But first we have to change some of our habits, which is the toughest thing to do in this whole affair.

Weight gain is a manifestation of harmful daily habits, and we lose weight when we change these habits. This is not easy. Our habits are the result of time and they are embedded in everything we do. Weight gain and harmful daily habits are so tightly bound together that to unravel one, we must untangle the other. If we want to improve our health, we have to be willing to modify what it is we've been doing.

This is scary.

I don't know anyone who doesn't find comfort in deeply rooted habits, however harmful or hindering they may be.

Losing weight long term is not for the faint of heart

It takes time, effort, and organization to undo our automatic and comfortable routines — from how we think about food, to how we shop, prepare, cook, and eat. No matter how important our reasons may be for losing weight, doing so demands a giant leap of faith, and a hefty dose of discipline.

We need discipline until we change the habit

A degree of discipline is certainly required at the start, along with a hearty dose of determination and diligence. But once the new habits set in, and the pounds start to fall off, energy levels will steadily increase. As the new habits become routine and enjoyable, reverting back to old ways becomes less appealing because we will like the way we now eat, move, and feel. Why would we want to carry a heavy suitcase or backpack with us, day in and day out, when we can settle into this simpler, lighter way of living? Here's our chance to unpack that unnecessary weight we've been lugging around with us for years and to start fresh with a clearer perspective and healthier habits.

A Few Strategies to Help Get the Brain On Board.

1. *Don't listen to Tinkerbell.*

   Block out the nagging voices telling us to ditch the whole thing, that we only live once, and why not just have fun. Most of them come from our own heads, so we can control them. Sometimes it's family and friends who found us to be more fun when we were willing to indulge. Don't fall for that. We know all too well where that rabbit hole leads — back to the beginning all over again!

Tinkerbell will taunt you with sweet temptations. That's her way. Sometimes your imaginary earplugs won't stay in, or you'll forget your blinders at home. Practise saying, "No, thanks." We all know those taunters and tempters, real or otherwise. Tell them to bother someone else.

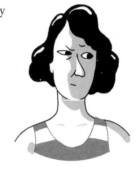

2. Be pragmatic.

You may know a few pragmatic people. I do. They assume there could be trouble. It never surprises them when it comes. They don't back away from it. A pragmatist is prepared for bad weather, which always strikes when a picnic is planned. Rather than wishing and hoping the day will be sunny and bright, they anticipate the storm, and are ready for it when it comes.

Taking a pragmatic approach to weight loss assures you'll be prepared for obstacles. And this time, when they do appear — and they always do — you won't pitch the diet in the trash and hope good intentions take you the rest of the way.

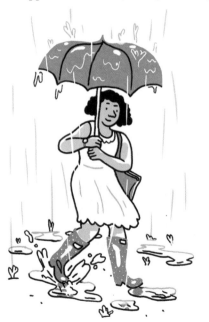

Half empty or half full?

Whichever way we look at it, losing weight is always about emptying the glass, however full or empty it may be. We can choose to see this task as arduous or easy, but regardless of our attitude towards it, weight loss still comes down to the same thing — emptying the stockroom less and exercising more.

It's the ones who stick it out, even in the face of resistance, who succeed. This is true for anything.

3. *Overcome your own resistance.*

Resistance is that pervasive and opposing force that lies within each one of us and prevents us from doing the work required to effect a positive change. Feeling resistance, however, does not mean we should revert back to our old ways just because they're comfortable. In time, being overweight won't be so comfortable.

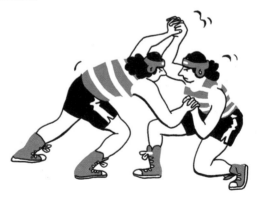

Resistance loves to sabotage.

Resistance is always waiting to pounce, especially when we embark on a long-term, life-altering venture such as this one. It rears its ugly head. We can fight against it, or we can let it knock us down and drag us back into the same patterns we've been trying to change for years.

Resistance is at its fiercest during weight loss because it is, by nature, impatient, and weight loss takes time. There's no realistic way to condense three months of minimizing into one. Resistance doesn't care for reality. It's terrified of change, no matter how important that change may be. It's always miserably comfortable with things exactly as they are.

We can try to understand and analyze resistance, but that won't help. We still have to override it. It lives within us. Our only choice is to fight it. Only we can stare it in the face and tell it to be quiet or get out of the way.

4. Recruit resilience.

Along with the resistance we all have within us, we have a greater stockpile of resilience waiting to be put to use. Resilience ploughs over impatience and self-pity. We can't skip over the time and effort that weight loss — or anything worthwhile — requires. Resilience recruits patience and perseverance. Even after the weight has been lost, perseverance is what prevents us from ravenously gobbling those pounds back on.

Resistance will continue to rear its ugly head, and resilience will have to keep right on smashing it back down again. Resilience has an element of wisdom running through it, because it knows, having tried and failed repeatedly, that reverting back to old habits only leads to refilling fat cells again. Resilience knows that we don't want to go back there again. Ever.

5. It's a lonely battle.

We're alone on this weight-loss quest. While we may not like this, it's the truth. It is, after all, our body, our brain, our life. No matter how much we may say we're doing it for our partners or our children, we're not. It's for ourselves. It had better be. Because this is a solitary battle.

Expecting the world around to congratulate us and cheer us on is a lot of pressure to put on other people, and will likely lead to disappointment. Neither friends nor family can ever offer the gratification we give ourselves for doing this. We must be steadfast in our conviction.

6. *Be prepared.*

When we understand the three principles and recruit the necessary mental strategies, it's time to get down to business. It is only by putting them into practice that we master them.

This means food. This means shopping. This means cooking.

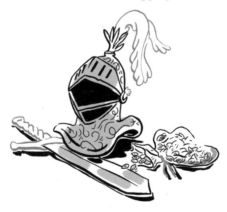

REVISE

When we stick to the principles, we'll lose the weight, and it will be easier than we ever imagined possible.

But then, suddenly, it will come to a screeching halt

Just when we think that the skies have finally opened up, and the pounds are falling away with unimaginable ease, things will squeal to a stop. Nothing will move. The scale may even start to tip the other way again. We must not panic.

Even if we're doing everything right, the body will always adapt. This is not a bad thing — it's just what it does. It means we have to shake things up.

Push through inertia

In the past, inertia may have got the better of us. This time, when we hit it, we'll be glad we know the principles and are no longer dieting blindly. We can employ strategies. We're savvy about the science now, so we can modify what we're doing — how we're eating and exercising.

The body will adapt to a reduction in calories, so we have to expect it. There's no way around this. It only makes sense that weight loss will slow down. If it didn't, there'd be a real problem. If our bodies didn't adapt, we'd eventually wither away to nothing. If we have more weight to lose, we need only revise slightly and the weight loss will continue.

Let's say we've been having a big salad every day for lunch for a while. It's full of good vegetables, a few nuts, half an avocado, olive oil, and vinegar — a blood sugar balancing bowl of goodness. It's only about 500 calories, but our weight loss has suddenly hit a standstill.

If we want to minimize further, without messing with blood sugar, we can switch to a soup instead. Make a big pot on the weekend with loads of vegetables and some chicken, seafood, or sausage, always starting with a tablespoon of olive oil. A bowl of soup at lunch will be half the calories of the salad — a difference of three pounds a month. If we need a bit more, we can have a few nuts, but if blood sugar is stable, we might find that a bowl of soup is sufficient. Details do matter at this point, but don't fret over it, just work with it.

Resistance is strongest at the end

We can overcome resistance at the start and we will have to overcome it again near the end. Resistance is always strongest at the end, just before we've conquered whatever battle we set out to win. Why? Because it loves to sabotage. Resistance will taunt us when it senses doubt. Don't give in to it. Revising is always a more worthwhile solution than quitting. It is never too late to tweak what we are doing. Now that we understand the principles, we don't need another diet and we also don't have to throw in the cards. We need only to revisit the principles and fit them in our daily habits in the most simple, strategic way possible.

If we've made it this far, we're on the right track. We will stay positive and modify. The smallest adjustment will keep that subtraction going. Continue to stabilize blood sugar, minimize further, get stronger, and walk longer. Ignite that fire, and keep burning those calories.

Whatever you do, don't sabotage your efforts now.

KEEP IT GOING!

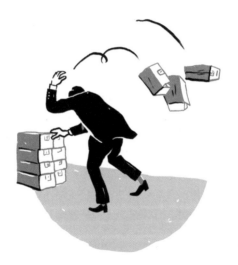

Acknowledgements

Many people have helped — in countless ways — bring this book from conception to completion.

Michael Bédard, Philip Sung, William Woods, Martha Butterfield, Shane Dolgin, Margaret Webb, Gerry Shikatani, Melanie Hazell, Chris Behnisch, Chris Willenberg, Marla Baker, Lindsay Angus, Kristen Ross, Sandra Richmond, and Connie Reeve — thank you for the astute edits and poignant suggestions.

Bjoern Arthurs — thank you for seeing the vision and bringing the analogies to life with brilliant illustrations.

Jeff Gosselin — thank you for believing in the idea and for supporting such an endeavour.

Finally, I am ever grateful to the men and women I work with who inspire me to uncover and clarify the essentials. Your questions, our conversations instil in me the impetus to decipher and simplify the complex science of the body, the brain, exercise, and food.

I hope this book provides needed clarity.